Macular Degeneration

Understanding Age-Related Vision Loss and Managing Symptoms

Eye Health, Early Detection, Treatment Options, Risk Factors, Improving Quality of Life, Vision Preservation Strategies and Lifestyle Adjustments for Better Vision

Graham Julian Oliver

Disclaimer

The information contained in this book, *Macular Degeneration - Understanding Age-Related Vision Loss and Managing Symptoms*, is intended for educational and informational purposes only. It is not intended as a substitute for professional medical advice, diagnosis, or treatment. Always seek the advice of your physician or other qualified health provider with any questions you may have regarding a medical condition or treatment.

The author does not provide any guarantees regarding the effectiveness or applicability of the information presented in this book. Individual results may vary, and the author assumes no responsibility for any actions taken based on the information provided in this book.

Furthermore, the author does not endorse any individual, product, website, organization, or other names mentioned within this book. References to specific products, services, or organizations are solely for informational purposes and do not imply any affiliation or endorsement.

About This Book

The book "Macular Degeneration - Understanding Age-Related Vision Loss and Managing Symptoms" serves as a crucial resource for individuals facing the challenges associated with macular degeneration. This condition is a leading cause of vision loss among older adults, significantly impacting their daily activities and overall quality of life. By providing a comprehensive overview of macular degeneration, including its definitions, types, and the anatomy of the eye, the book emphasizes the importance of understanding this condition. It addresses how macular degeneration specifically affects central vision, which is essential for tasks such as reading and driving, thus highlighting the necessity for early detection and effective management strategies.

In addition to elucidating the fundamental aspects of macular degeneration, the book delves into the critical significance of eye health. The macula, a small but vital part of the retina, plays a crucial role in our vision. The text articulates how maintaining eye health is closely linked to overall well-being, underscoring the importance of regular eye exams for early diagnosis and intervention. With advancements in treatment options and lifestyle modifications, readers are empowered to take proactive steps toward preserving their vision. These insights create a foundation for understanding not just the clinical aspects of the disease, but also the emotional and psychological challenges it presents.

The exploration of treatment options is particularly vital, as it provides a detailed overview of available therapies, including nutritional supplements and anti-VEGF injections for wet macular degeneration. By emphasizing the importance of personalized treatment plans, the book equips readers with knowledge about their choices and encourages collaboration with healthcare professionals. Moreover, the discussion of innovative technologies and emerging therapies keeps readers informed about the latest advancements in the field, ensuring they remain hopeful and engaged in their care.

Risk factors for macular degeneration, such as age, genetic predisposition, and lifestyle choices, are critically examined to help readers assess their personal risk profiles. Understanding these factors is pivotal in implementing preventive measures that can significantly reduce the likelihood of developing the condition. The text also stresses the role of public health awareness and education in risk management, highlighting the need for community engagement in promoting eye health.

Enhancing quality of life for individuals experiencing vision loss is another key focus of this book. It provides practical strategies for coping with vision challenges, including the use of assistive devices and the importance of support groups. By fostering an environment of understanding and adaptation, the book addresses the emotional aspects of living with macular degeneration and emphasizes the vital role of family and caregivers in this journey. This holistic approach ensures that readers not only navigate the technicalities of their condition but also cultivate resilience and maintain their independence.

To further support readers, the book outlines vision preservation strategies through nutritional advice and lifestyle adjustments. By encouraging the consumption of eye-healthy foods, regular exercise, and protective measures against UV rays, it provides actionable tips for improving and maintaining eye health. Moreover, the book emphasizes the significance of routine eye care and creating an eye-friendly environment, allowing individuals to take control of their vision health proactively.

The discussion around common concerns related to macular degeneration addresses the fears and misconceptions that often accompany a diagnosis. By providing clear, factual information and strategies for open communication, the book helps demystify the condition and supports readers in managing their emotional and financial concerns effectively. It also fosters a sense of community among individuals facing similar challenges, encouraging connections and shared experiences.

Lastly, the FAQs section serves as a valuable resource for readers, addressing common inquiries about macular degeneration and offering insights into current research advancements. By presenting a comprehensive and accessible guide, **"Macular Degeneration - Understanding Age-Related Vision Loss and Managing Symptoms"** not only empowers individuals affected by the condition but also serves as a beacon of hope, encouraging them to prioritize their eye health and seek the support they need for a fulfilling life.

Table of Contents

Introduction

Definition of Macular Degeneration

Macular degeneration, also known as age-related macular degeneration (AMD), is a medical condition that affects the macula, the central part of the retina responsible for sharp, detailed vision. It leads to the gradual deterioration of the macula, resulting in a decline in visual acuity, particularly in the central field of vision. Understanding this condition is crucial for early intervention and management.

This vision disorder primarily affects individuals over the age of 50, making it vital for this age group to be aware of the signs and symptoms. Early detection can help slow down the progression of the disease and preserve remaining vision. Regular eye exams and awareness of changes in vision can aid in recognizing the onset of macular degeneration.

Overview of Its Significance as a Leading Cause of Vision Loss in Older Adults

Macular degeneration is a significant public health concern as it stands as one of the leading causes of vision loss among older adults. It can profoundly impact an individual's ability to perform daily tasks, such as reading, driving, and recognizing faces, severely affecting their quality of life. Awareness of this condition's prevalence emphasizes the need for preventive measures and timely treatment.

The significance of addressing macular degeneration lies not only in preserving vision but also in maintaining independence and mental well-being among older adults. The emotional and social implications of vision loss can lead to isolation and depression. Thus, recognizing macular degeneration's impact highlights the importance of comprehensive eye care in aging populations.

The Impact of the Condition on Daily Life and Activities

The effects of macular degeneration on daily life can be profound, making it challenging to engage in activities that require clear central vision. Tasks like reading, cooking, and watching television may become increasingly difficult, leading to frustration and dependence on others. The gradual loss of independence can significantly alter an individual's lifestyle and mental health.

Moreover, the inability to recognize faces or read street signs can lead to anxiety and reduced confidence when navigating familiar environments. Many individuals with macular degeneration may also experience difficulties in driving, further limiting their independence. Understanding these impacts can guide families and caregivers in providing the necessary support and resources.

The Importance of Understanding Risk Factors and Preventive Measures

Recognizing the risk factors associated with macular degeneration is essential for prevention and early detection. Key factors include age, genetics, smoking, obesity, and prolonged exposure to sunlight. Individuals should be proactive by discussing their risk factors with an eye care professional and getting regular eye exams, especially if they have a family history of the disease.

Preventive measures can include adopting a healthy lifestyle, such as a balanced diet rich in leafy greens and omega-3 fatty acids, maintaining a healthy weight, and quitting smoking. Regular exercise can also play a crucial role in reducing the risk of macular degeneration. By understanding and addressing these risk factors, individuals can significantly decrease their chances of developing this vision-threatening condition.

Brief Mention of the Different Types (Dry and Wet) of Macular Degeneration

Macular degeneration primarily presents in two forms: dry and wet. Dry macular degeneration is the most common type, accounting for about 80-90% of cases. It involves the gradual thinning of the macula, leading to a slow loss of vision over time. Patients with dry AMD often notice blurriness or difficulty in reading, and while it progresses slowly, it can eventually lead to significant vision loss.

Wet macular degeneration, while less common, is more severe and can lead to rapid vision loss. It occurs when abnormal blood vessels grow under the retina and leak fluid or blood, causing scarring and distortion in vision. Early treatment options, such as anti-VEGF injections, can help manage this form of AMD and preserve vision. Understanding these types aids in recognizing symptoms early and seeking appropriate medical care.

Importance of Eye Health

Explanation of the Macula's Role in Vision

The macula is a small, highly sensitive area located in the center of the retina, responsible for our sharpest and most detailed vision. It enables us to perform tasks that require fine vision, such as reading, driving, and recognizing faces. The macula contains a high concentration of photoreceptor cells, called cones, which are essential for color perception and central vision.

Understanding the macula's function is crucial, as damage to this area can lead to significant vision problems. When the macula deteriorates, it can impair the ability to see fine details, affecting daily activities. Knowing how the macula works can motivate individuals to prioritize eye health and seek regular check-ups.

How Macular Degeneration Affects Central Vision

Macular degeneration primarily affects central vision, leading to challenges in tasks that rely on sharp eyesight. Individuals may experience blurred or distorted vision, making it difficult to read or recognize faces. In advanced stages, a dark or empty spot may develop in the center of the visual field, significantly impacting quality of life.

It's essential to note that while macular degeneration does not lead to complete blindness, it can severely limit independence and daily functioning. Recognizing early symptoms can prompt individuals to seek medical advice sooner, potentially slowing the progression of the disease.

The Relationship between Eye Health and Overall Well-Being

Eye health is closely linked to overall well-being, as good vision is essential for maintaining independence and quality of life. Poor eye health can lead to various complications, such as difficulty in performing daily tasks, increased risk of falls, and reduced social interactions, all of which can negatively impact mental health.

Maintaining eye health involves adopting a comprehensive approach, including proper nutrition, regular exercise, and managing chronic conditions like diabetes and hypertension. By prioritizing eye health, individuals can enhance their overall well-being and prevent vision-related challenges.

The Significance of Regular Eye Exams for Early Detection

Regular eye exams are vital for the early detection of macular degeneration and other eye conditions. During an eye exam, an eye care professional can assess the health of the retina and identify any changes that may indicate the onset of macular degeneration. Early detection is crucial as it allows for timely intervention, which can help slow disease progression.

For optimal eye health, adults should have comprehensive eye exams at least every one to two years, or more frequently if risk factors are present. Keeping track of vision changes and discussing any concerns with a healthcare provider can significantly improve outcomes.

Overview of Advancements in Treatment Options and Lifestyle Modifications

Recent advancements in treatment options for macular degeneration include anti-VEGF injections, laser therapy, and photodynamic therapy, which aim to slow disease progression and preserve vision. These treatments target the underlying causes of macular degeneration, such as abnormal blood vessel growth, and can help stabilize vision for many patients.

In addition to medical treatments, lifestyle modifications play a critical role in managing macular degeneration. Eating a diet rich in leafy greens, fish, and antioxidants, along with engaging in regular physical activity, can support eye health. These adjustments can significantly improve quality of life and promote better vision outcomes.

CHAPTER 1:

Understanding Macular Degeneration

Definition and Types (Dry and Wet)

Macular degeneration (MD) is a progressive eye condition affecting the macula, the central part of the retina responsible for sharp vision. There are two primary types: **dry** macular degeneration, which is more common and occurs when the light-sensitive cells in the macula break down, leading to gradual vision loss; and **wet** macular degeneration, which involves the growth of abnormal blood vessels beneath the retina, causing rapid and severe vision impairment. Understanding these types is crucial for determining appropriate treatment and management strategies.

To manage MD effectively, it's essential to recognize which type you or a loved one has. Regular eye exams can help in early detection, and lifestyle changes can support overall eye health. For dry MD, nutritional supplements, such as those containing lutein and zeaxanthin, may slow progression. In contrast, wet MD might require medical interventions like anti-VEGF injections to control abnormal blood vessel growth.

Causes and Risk Factors

The causes of macular degeneration are multifactorial, involving a combination of genetic, environmental, and lifestyle factors. Age is the most significant risk factor, with the condition typically developing in individuals over 50. Other factors include a family history of MD, smoking, obesity, and exposure to sunlight, which can increase oxidative stress in the eyes.

To minimize the risk, individuals should focus on lifestyle changes such as quitting smoking, maintaining a healthy weight, and wearing UV-blocking sunglasses outdoors. Regular check-ups with an eye care professional can help monitor risk factors and ensure early intervention if MD begins to develop.

The Anatomy of the Eye and the Role of the Macula

Understanding the anatomy of the eye is vital for grasping the impact of macular degeneration. The eye consists of several parts, including the cornea, lens, retina, and the macula, which is located in the center of the retina. The macula is crucial for central vision, allowing us to see fine details clearly, essential for tasks like reading and recognizing faces.

To maintain eye health, it's important to protect and care for the macula. This can be achieved by consuming a diet rich in leafy greens and fish, which provide essential nutrients like omega-3 fatty acids and antioxidants. Regular eye exams are also key, as they can help detect changes in the macula early, allowing for timely intervention.

How Age Affects Eye Health

As we age, our eyes undergo various changes that can impact vision quality. The lens may become less flexible, leading to conditions such as presbyopia, while the retina can become thinner, increasing the risk of age-related diseases, including macular degeneration. These changes can affect the way we see colors and details, making it harder to perform everyday tasks.

To combat age-related vision decline, individuals should adopt habits that promote eye health. This includes a balanced diet, staying hydrated, and incorporating regular physical activity to improve circulation. Additionally, managing chronic conditions like diabetes and hypertension can help reduce the risk of age-related vision problems.

Symptoms and Stages of Macular Degeneration

Symptoms of macular degeneration can vary based on its stage. Early stages may show no noticeable symptoms, while more advanced stages can cause blurred vision, difficulty reading, and distorted images. Individuals might notice straight lines appearing wavy or having dark or empty spots in their central vision.

To monitor symptoms effectively, maintaining an Amsler grid at home can help individuals detect changes in their vision. Regular consultations with an eye care professional are crucial for assessing the condition's progression and adjusting treatment plans as needed.

Differences between Macular Degeneration and Other Eye Diseases

Macular degeneration often gets confused with other eye diseases, such as glaucoma and cataracts, but they affect different parts of the eye and have distinct symptoms. While glaucoma involves increased pressure in the eye leading to peripheral vision loss, cataracts cause clouding of the lens, affecting overall vision clarity. Understanding these differences is important for proper diagnosis and treatment.

To differentiate between these conditions, it's essential to undergo comprehensive eye examinations, which can include visual acuity tests and imaging techniques. Being aware of the unique symptoms associated with each condition can empower individuals to seek appropriate care and treatment.

Genetic Factors Influencing Macular Degeneration

Genetic factors play a significant role in the risk of developing macular degeneration. Specific genes, such as the CFH and ARMS2 genes, have been linked to an increased risk of both dry and wet forms of MD. If there is a family history of macular degeneration, individuals may have a higher likelihood of developing the condition themselves.

To address genetic risks, individuals can consider genetic testing if there is a strong family history of MD. Furthermore, discussing family history with an eye care professional can lead to more personalized monitoring and preventive strategies, including lifestyle modifications that may reduce risk.

Common Myths and Misconceptions

Several myths surround macular degeneration that can lead to misunderstandings about the condition. One common misconception is that MD only affects older adults, while it can also occur in younger individuals, particularly if they have specific genetic risk factors. Another myth is that once vision loss occurs, nothing can be done, but there are treatments and lifestyle changes that can help slow progression and improve quality of life.

To combat misinformation, it's essential to seek out credible sources of information regarding macular degeneration. Engaging with eye care professionals and participating in educational programs can help individuals and families better understand the condition and its management options.

The Role of Oxidative Stress in Eye Health

Oxidative stress refers to the damage caused by free radicals, which can lead to cellular damage in the eye and contribute to the development of macular degeneration. Factors such as smoking, poor diet, and environmental toxins can increase oxidative stress, adversely affecting eye health.

To reduce oxidative stress, individuals should focus on incorporating antioxidants into their diet through foods like berries, nuts, and green vegetables. Additionally, reducing exposure to environmental toxins and avoiding smoking can significantly benefit overall eye health and may help mitigate the risk of developing macular degeneration.

Importance of Early Detection

Early detection of macular degeneration is critical in managing the disease effectively. Regular eye exams can help identify changes in vision before significant damage occurs, allowing for timely intervention and treatment. Detecting MD in its early stages can significantly affect the long-term prognosis and quality of life.

To facilitate early detection, individuals should prioritize routine eye exams, especially if they are over 50 or have risk factors for macular degeneration. Keeping a record of any changes in vision and discussing them with an eye care professional can also lead to prompt evaluation and necessary action.

Current Statistics on Prevalence

Macular degeneration is one of the leading causes of vision loss among older adults, affecting millions worldwide. According to current statistics, approximately 10 million Americans have some form of age-related macular degeneration, with prevalence expected to rise as the population ages. Understanding these statistics highlights the importance of awareness and proactive management of eye health.

To combat the rising prevalence, community education and outreach are essential. Individuals can participate in local health fairs or seminars focused on eye health to learn more about prevention, early detection, and available treatment options for macular degeneration.

The Emotional Impact of Vision Loss

The emotional impact of vision loss due to macular degeneration can be significant, leading to feelings of frustration, sadness, and anxiety. Individuals may struggle with the loss of independence and changes in daily activities, which can affect their mental health and overall well-being. It's essential to acknowledge these feelings and seek support.

To manage emotional challenges, individuals should consider joining support groups where they can share experiences and coping strategies with others facing similar challenges. Engaging with mental health professionals can also provide valuable tools for navigating the emotional aspects of vision loss.

Future Research Directions

Research on macular degeneration continues to evolve, focusing on better understanding its underlying mechanisms and developing innovative treatments. Current studies are exploring gene therapy, new medications, and potential surgical options to treat and manage both dry and wet forms of the disease. Keeping abreast of advancements in research is vital for individuals at risk.

To stay informed, individuals should engage with reputable organizations dedicated to eye health and subscribe to relevant journals or newsletters. Participating in clinical trials can also provide access to cutting-edge treatments while contributing to the broader understanding of macular degeneration.

CHAPTER 2:

Early Detection and Diagnosis

Importance of Regular Eye Exams

Regular eye exams are crucial for detecting early signs of macular degeneration and other vision issues. These exams allow eye care professionals to assess your eye health and monitor any changes over time. Ideally, individuals over 50 should schedule comprehensive eye exams at least once a year, as early detection can significantly improve treatment outcomes.

During these exams, optometrists or ophthalmologists evaluate not just vision but also the overall health of your eyes. They look for changes in the retina and other structures that may indicate macular degeneration. Being proactive about eye exams ensures any potential issues are caught early, allowing for timely intervention and management.

Common Diagnostic Tests (e.g., Amsler Grid, OCT)

Common diagnostic tests used to assess macular degeneration include the Amsler grid and Optical Coherence Tomography (OCT). The Amsler grid is a simple tool that you can use at home to monitor your vision. By focusing on the center dot and noting any distortions or blind spots, you can track changes and report them to your eye care provider.

OCT is a non-invasive imaging test that provides detailed images of the retina. During the test, you'll place your chin on a rest while the machine scans your eyes. This allows your doctor to evaluate the layers of the retina and identify any abnormalities associated with macular degeneration, aiding in early detection and appropriate treatment planning.

Signs to Watch for at Home

Being vigilant about your vision can help you identify early signs of macular degeneration. Look out for symptoms like blurred or distorted vision, difficulty recognizing faces, or a gradual loss of central vision. Keeping a journal of any changes can help communicate your observations to your healthcare provider.

You can also use tools like the Amsler grid at home to regularly check for visual distortions. If you notice any changes, it's essential to schedule an appointment with your eye care professional as soon as possible to assess your eye health and determine next steps.

Role of Family History in Monitoring Risk

Family history plays a significant role in assessing your risk for macular degeneration. If you have relatives with the condition, it's important to inform your eye care provider, as genetic factors can increase your likelihood of developing the disease. Understanding your family history can guide the frequency of eye exams and the need for monitoring.

Being aware of your family's eye health can also help you adopt preventive measures. Discussing any known conditions with family members and encouraging them to get regular eye check-ups can create a proactive approach to managing vision health across generations.

How Optometrists and Ophthalmologists Diagnose the Condition

Optometrists and ophthalmologists use a combination of patient history, visual acuity tests, and imaging to diagnose macular degeneration. During your visit, the doctor will ask about your symptoms, family history, and any changes in your vision. This information is crucial for forming a complete picture of your eye health.

After the initial assessment, eye care professionals may conduct additional tests, including dilation to examine the retina and specialized imaging tests like OCT. These procedures help confirm the diagnosis and determine the most appropriate treatment options based on the severity and type of macular degeneration.

The Significance of Visual Acuity Tests

Visual acuity tests are essential for assessing how well you see at various distances. During the test, you'll read letters from a chart, helping your eye care provider evaluate the clarity of your vision. Regular testing can reveal changes in visual acuity, which may indicate the progression of macular degeneration.

Maintaining a record of your visual acuity over time allows for better monitoring of your condition. If you notice a decline in your ability to see clearly, it's important to discuss these changes with your eye care professional, who can suggest further testing or modifications to your management plan.

Importance of Discussing Symptoms with Healthcare Providers

Open communication with your healthcare provider about any vision changes is vital for effective management of macular degeneration. Discuss any symptoms, such as blurriness, blind spots, or difficulty seeing in low light. Being honest and detailed about your experiences helps your provider tailor a monitoring and treatment plan specifically for you.

Don't hesitate to ask questions or seek clarification about your diagnosis and treatment options. Understanding your condition can empower you to take an active role in managing your eye health and make informed decisions regarding any necessary lifestyle adjustments.

Referral Processes to Specialists

If your eye care provider suspects advanced macular degeneration, they may refer you to a specialist, such as a retinal surgeon. This referral process often involves sharing your medical records and diagnostic test results to ensure a seamless transition for your care. Your provider will discuss the next steps and what to expect during your appointment with the specialist.

Once referred, the specialist will perform further evaluations and may recommend specific treatment options. Being proactive about follow-up appointments and discussing any additional concerns with your primary provider will help maintain continuity in your care.

Monitoring Progression Over Time

Monitoring the progression of macular degeneration is crucial for effective management. Regular follow-up appointments with your eye care provider will help assess any changes in your condition. Your doctor may schedule more frequent visits if they notice significant progression or if you experience new symptoms.

Keep track of any changes in your vision and report them during your appointments. Documenting your experiences can provide valuable insights into how your condition is evolving, aiding your provider in making informed decisions about your treatment and management strategies.

Emerging Diagnostic Technologies

Emerging diagnostic technologies are enhancing the ability to detect and manage macular degeneration. Innovations such as advanced imaging techniques and genetic testing offer more precise assessments of the condition. These technologies help identify patients at risk and tailor treatment options to individual needs.

Stay informed about these advancements by discussing them with your eye care provider. They can guide you on the most current technologies available and how they may apply to your situation, ensuring you receive the best possible care.

What to Expect During an Eye Exam

During an eye exam for macular degeneration, expect a comprehensive assessment of your vision and eye health. The process typically includes visual acuity tests, dilation, and possibly imaging techniques like OCT. You may be asked about your symptoms and family history to help guide the evaluation.

Dilation involves the use of eye drops to widen your pupils, allowing your doctor to see the retina more clearly. While your vision may be blurry for a short time afterward, this step is essential for a thorough examination. Your eye care provider will explain each part of the process and what findings may indicate regarding your eye health.

The Role of Community Awareness Programs

Community awareness programs play a vital role in educating the public about macular degeneration and promoting proactive eye health practices. These initiatives often include workshops, seminars, and informational resources that help individuals understand the importance of early detection and regular eye exams.

Participating in community programs can enhance your knowledge of macular degeneration, including risk factors and management strategies. Engaging with these resources fosters a supportive environment where you can learn from professionals and connect with others facing similar challenges.

Encouraging Proactive Eye Health Practices

Encouraging proactive eye health practices is key to preventing and managing macular degeneration. This includes scheduling regular eye exams, eating a balanced diet rich in antioxidants, and protecting your eyes from UV rays with sunglasses. Simple lifestyle changes, like quitting smoking and maintaining a healthy weight, can also lower your risk.

Education about eye health should start early and continue throughout life. Share information with family and friends, emphasizing the importance of routine check-ups and healthy habits. By fostering a culture of awareness, you can help others take charge of their eye health and mitigate the risk of vision loss.

CHAPTER 3:

Treatment Options

Overview of Available Treatments

Macular degeneration is primarily treated through a variety of methods tailored to the type and severity of the condition. For dry macular degeneration, available treatments include nutritional supplements and lifestyle changes to slow progression. Wet macular degeneration often requires more intensive interventions, such as injections or laser therapies. Understanding these options can help patients and caregivers make informed decisions.

Consultation with an eye care specialist is crucial to identify the most suitable treatment for individual cases. Regular monitoring and adjustments based on progression and response to treatments can enhance outcomes. A well-rounded approach that combines various treatment modalities often yields the best results for managing macular degeneration.

Nutritional Supplements and Their Role (AREDS Formula)

The Age-Related Eye Disease Study (AREDS) established that specific nutritional supplements can significantly impact the progression of macular degeneration. The AREDS formula typically includes antioxidants like vitamins C and E, zinc, and copper, which are believed to help protect retinal cells from damage. Incorporating these supplements into your daily routine may slow the progression of the disease.

To effectively utilize the AREDS formula, consult your healthcare provider for personalized recommendations. It's essential to choose high-quality supplements that contain the appropriate dosages as recommended by AREDS. Combining these with a balanced diet rich in leafy greens, fish, and nuts can enhance their protective effects on eye health.

Anti-VEGF Injections for Wet Macular Degeneration

Anti-VEGF (vascular endothelial growth factor) injections are a cornerstone treatment for wet macular degeneration. These injections work by blocking the growth of abnormal blood vessels that can leak fluid and cause vision loss. Typically administered every four to eight weeks, these injections can stabilize or even improve vision for many patients.

For effective treatment, it's important to schedule regular appointments with your ophthalmologist. They will assess the condition of your macula and determine the appropriate timing and frequency of injections. Understanding the process can help reduce anxiety about the procedure, which is relatively quick and involves minimal discomfort.

Photodynamic Therapy Explained

Photodynamic therapy (PDT) is another innovative treatment option for wet macular degeneration. This technique involves administering a light-sensitive drug that targets abnormal blood vessels in the eye. Once the drug is injected, a specific wavelength of light is applied to activate the medication, effectively sealing off the leaking vessels and preventing further vision loss.

To undergo PDT, patients should follow pre-treatment guidelines, which may include avoiding sunlight and bright indoor lights for a specified period after the treatment. Discussing potential side effects and the number of sessions required with your eye care professional can help set expectations and ensure a smoother treatment process.

Laser Therapy as a Treatment Option

Laser therapy utilizes focused light to target and destroy abnormal blood vessels in the retina associated with wet macular degeneration. This method can help preserve vision and prevent further deterioration. Laser treatments can be administered in a single session, but multiple treatments may be needed depending on individual circumstances.

Before undergoing laser therapy, patients should understand the procedure and what to expect during recovery. It's essential to follow post-treatment care instructions provided by the healthcare provider to optimize healing and minimize complications.

Vision Rehabilitation Services

Vision rehabilitation services are designed to help individuals cope with vision loss caused by macular degeneration. These services may include occupational therapy, mobility training, and the use of assistive devices to enhance daily functioning. A personalized rehabilitation plan can help improve independence and quality of life.

Engaging with a certified vision rehabilitation specialist can provide tailored strategies to navigate visual challenges. This may involve learning how to use specialized tools, such as magnifiers or electronic devices, effectively. Regular participation in these services can lead to improved confidence and adaptability in daily activities.

The Importance of Personalized Treatment Plans

Every individual's experience with macular degeneration is unique, necessitating personalized treatment plans. Factors such as the type of macular degeneration, overall health, and personal preferences should be considered when developing a management strategy. This personalized approach can significantly enhance treatment effectiveness and patient satisfaction.

Patients should work closely with their healthcare providers to create and adjust their treatment plans. Regular check-ins to discuss progress, side effects, and new symptoms can lead to timely modifications in treatment, ensuring the best possible outcomes.

Clinical Trials and Emerging Therapies

Participating in clinical trials can provide access to cutting-edge therapies for macular degeneration that may not yet be widely available. These trials are critical for advancing treatment options and may offer patients new hope for improved vision. Eligibility criteria and the potential benefits or risks of participating in trials should be thoroughly discussed with a healthcare professional.

For those considering participation, researching ongoing trials and discussing options with an ophthalmologist can provide valuable insights. It's essential to weigh the potential benefits against the uncertainties, ensuring that informed decisions are made regarding participation.

The Role of Innovative Technologies in Treatment

Innovative technologies are transforming the treatment landscape for macular degeneration. Advancements such as telemedicine, digital imaging, and home monitoring devices allow for earlier detection and more effective management. These technologies facilitate remote consultations and regular monitoring, helping patients maintain their vision while reducing the need for frequent in-person visits.

To make the most of these technological advancements, patients should stay informed about the latest options available. Discussing the use of specific devices or apps with eye care professionals can enhance the management of macular degeneration and empower patients to take an active role in their care.

Collaboration with Healthcare Professionals

Effective management of macular degeneration requires collaboration among various healthcare professionals, including ophthalmologists, optometrists, nutritionists, and rehabilitation specialists. This team approach ensures that all aspects of a patient's health and vision are addressed comprehensively. Regular communication among the team members helps streamline care and optimize treatment outcomes.

Patients should actively participate in this collaborative process by sharing their experiences and concerns with their healthcare team. Establishing clear communication pathways can lead to better coordination of care and a more holistic approach to managing macular degeneration.

Cost Considerations and Insurance Coverage

Understanding the costs associated with macular degeneration treatments is essential for effective management. Many treatment options, such as injections or therapies, can be expensive, and patients should check their insurance coverage to identify what is included. Discussing payment options and financial assistance programs with healthcare providers can help alleviate some of the financial burdens.

Patients are encouraged to advocate for their needs by asking about the costs and insurance implications before initiating any treatment. Exploring community resources and support groups can also provide additional assistance in navigating the financial aspects of care.

The Impact of Treatments on Quality of Life

The effectiveness of macular degeneration treatments can significantly influence a patient's quality of life. Many treatments aim not only to preserve vision but also to improve daily functioning and overall well-being. Understanding the potential benefits and limitations of each treatment can help patients set realistic expectations for their vision and lifestyle.

Regular follow-ups with healthcare providers to assess the impact of treatments on daily activities and emotional well-being are crucial. This feedback can lead to necessary adjustments in treatment plans, ensuring that patients maintain the best possible quality of life throughout their journey with macular degeneration.

Staying Informed About New Developments in Treatment

Staying informed about new treatments and research developments in macular degeneration is vital for patients. Emerging therapies, clinical trial results, and advancements in technology can provide new hope for improved vision and management strategies. Patients should actively seek information through reputable sources, such as healthcare providers and specialized organizations.

Engaging with support groups and online communities can also facilitate knowledge sharing among individuals facing similar challenges. By staying informed, patients can make educated decisions about their treatment options and advocate effectively for their needs.

CHAPTER 4:

Risk Factors for Macular Degeneration

Age and its Correlation with Risk

As individuals age, the risk of developing age-related macular degeneration (AMD) significantly increases. The macula, which is the central part of the retina responsible for sharp vision, undergoes changes that can lead to deterioration over time. By age 50, the likelihood of AMD begins to rise, and it becomes more prevalent in those over 70. Regular eye examinations are essential to monitor changes in vision and detect any early signs of macular degeneration.

To mitigate risk associated with age, it is crucial to adopt a proactive approach to eye health. This includes scheduling annual comprehensive eye exams, as early detection can lead to more effective management of AMD. Additionally, individuals should be aware of the normal age-related changes in vision, such as difficulty reading small print, to recognize when it may be time to consult a healthcare professional.

Genetic Predisposition and Family History

Genetic factors play a significant role in the development of AMD, with family history being a key indicator of risk. If someone has a parent or sibling with AMD, their chances of developing the condition increase significantly. Genetic testing may provide insights into one's susceptibility, allowing for informed decisions regarding monitoring and preventive measures.

Understanding family history is vital for assessing personal risk. Individuals with a known family history of AMD should discuss this with their eye care provider, who can recommend appropriate screening schedules. Awareness of genetic predispositions can encourage proactive measures, such as lifestyle modifications and regular check-ups, to potentially delay the onset of symptoms.

Lifestyle Factors: Smoking and Diet

Smoking is one of the most significant modifiable risk factors for AMD. Research shows that smokers are at a higher risk of developing the disease than non-smokers. Quitting smoking can greatly reduce the risk and improve overall eye health. To support this change, individuals can seek help through support groups or cessation programs that provide resources and strategies for quitting.

Diet also plays a crucial role in managing the risk of AMD. Consuming a diet rich in leafy greens, colorful fruits, and omega-3 fatty acids can promote eye health. Incorporating foods like spinach, kale, and fish into daily meals can provide essential nutrients that may help preserve vision. Keeping a food diary to track dietary habits can help individuals identify areas for improvement and make healthier choices.

The Role of Obesity and Physical Activity

Obesity is linked to an increased risk of developing AMD due to its association with inflammation and poor circulation. Maintaining a healthy weight through balanced nutrition and regular exercise can lower this risk. Engaging in physical activity, such as walking, swimming, or cycling, not only supports weight management but also promotes overall cardiovascular health, benefiting the eyes.

To effectively manage weight, individuals can set realistic goals and incorporate physical activity into their daily routines. Simple changes, like taking the stairs instead of the elevator or walking during lunch breaks, can contribute to a more active lifestyle. Tracking physical activity with apps or fitness trackers can help motivate individuals to stay consistent and monitor their progress.

Sun Exposure and Blue Light Effects

Excessive sun exposure can damage the retina and increase the risk of AMD. Wearing sunglasses with UV protection when outdoors is essential to shield the eyes from harmful rays. Choosing sunglasses that block 100% of UVA and UVB rays can provide significant protection. It's also advisable to wear a wide-brimmed hat for additional coverage.

Additionally, blue light from digital devices has raised concerns regarding eye health. To minimize exposure, individuals can use screen filters or enable blue light reduction settings on devices. Taking regular breaks from screens, following the 20-20-20 rule (looking at something 20 feet away for 20 seconds every 20 minutes), can also reduce eye strain and promote better visual comfort.

Other Health Conditions (e.g., Diabetes, Hypertension)

Chronic health conditions such as diabetes and hypertension can significantly impact eye health and increase the risk of AMD. High blood sugar levels in diabetics can lead to damage in the retina, making regular eye exams crucial for early detection and management. Individuals with these conditions should work closely with healthcare providers to monitor and control their health.

Managing blood sugar and blood pressure through medication, diet, and lifestyle changes can help reduce the risk of developing AMD. Maintaining a balanced diet low in sugar and sodium, along with regular physical activity, can support overall health. Individuals should keep a log of their health metrics to identify trends and areas needing improvement, which can be shared with healthcare providers for tailored advice.

Gender Differences in Prevalence

Research indicates that women are more likely to develop AMD than men, partly due to their longer life expectancy. Hormonal differences may also contribute to this increased risk. Understanding this disparity can prompt women to prioritize regular eye exams, particularly as they age, to catch any changes early.

To address this risk, women should educate themselves about AMD and discuss any concerns with their eye care professionals. Establishing a routine for eye examinations can help monitor vision changes, and women can benefit from participating in awareness programs focused on age-related eye health.

Ethnic Background and Susceptibility

Certain ethnic groups, particularly Caucasians, have a higher risk of developing AMD compared to others. Awareness of these trends can help individuals understand their personal risk and the importance of early detection. Ethnic background can influence access to healthcare and health education, so it's essential for those at higher risk to prioritize eye care.

Individuals from high-risk ethnic groups should actively seek information and resources regarding AMD. Engaging with community health programs or organizations can provide support and increase awareness of preventive measures. Taking part in local health screenings can also facilitate early detection and intervention, ultimately preserving vision.

How to Assess Personal Risk Factors

Assessing personal risk factors for AMD involves understanding both genetic and lifestyle influences. Individuals should consider their family history, lifestyle choices, and existing health conditions. Keeping a detailed health history can aid discussions with eye care professionals, who can then recommend appropriate screening based on assessed risks.

A personal risk assessment can also involve evaluating daily habits, such as diet, exercise, and sun exposure. Individuals can create a checklist of their risk factors to guide discussions with healthcare providers. Regularly reviewing and updating this list can help track changes and maintain a proactive approach to eye health.

Preventive Measures to Reduce Risk

Preventive measures to lower the risk of AMD include adopting a healthy lifestyle, such as quitting smoking, maintaining a balanced diet, and engaging in regular exercise. Regular eye exams are vital for early detection and management of any vision changes. Utilizing protective eyewear and following a healthy diet rich in antioxidants can further reduce risk.

In addition to personal measures, community awareness and education about AMD can lead to better prevention strategies. Individuals should participate in local health initiatives and support groups that promote eye health. By sharing information and resources, communities can collectively work toward reducing the impact of AMD on their populations.

Importance of Public Health Awareness

Public health awareness plays a crucial role in educating communities about AMD and its risk factors. Campaigns that promote eye health can lead to increased screening and early detection rates. By highlighting the importance of regular eye exams and lifestyle modifications, communities can foster a culture of prevention and proactive health management.

Engaging in public health initiatives, such as local health fairs or awareness campaigns, can empower individuals to take charge of their eye health. Schools and workplaces can also play a role in disseminating information about AMD, ensuring that people are informed about the risks and encouraged to seek regular check-ups.

The Role of Education in Risk Management

Education is a powerful tool in managing the risk of AMD. By understanding the disease, its risk factors, and preventive measures, individuals can make informed decisions about their eye health. Health education programs can provide vital information on lifestyle changes and screening recommendations to those at risk.

To maximize the benefits of education, individuals should seek out workshops, webinars, or community seminars focused on eye health. Accessing credible resources and sharing knowledge with friends and family can create a supportive environment that promotes awareness and encourages proactive measures to protect vision.

Recommendations for At-Risk Individuals

At-risk individuals for AMD should prioritize regular eye examinations to monitor for early signs of the disease. Staying informed about personal risk factors and engaging in preventive measures is essential. Eye care professionals may recommend supplements containing vitamins C and E, zinc, and lutein to support eye health.

Developing a comprehensive plan that includes lifestyle modifications, such as a balanced diet and regular physical activity, can enhance overall well-being.

CHAPTER 5:

Improving Quality of Life

Strategies for Coping with Vision Loss

Coping with vision loss requires a proactive approach to maintain quality of life. One effective strategy is to develop a routine that accommodates changes in vision, allowing for better predictability in daily activities. This can include using consistent locations for items and organizing spaces to minimize confusion. Engaging in relaxation techniques such as meditation can also help manage the emotional impact of vision loss, enabling individuals to approach challenges with a more positive mindset.

Additionally, learning to focus on remaining abilities rather than limitations can foster resilience. This involves setting realistic goals and celebrating small achievements, which can enhance motivation and overall well-being. Support from healthcare professionals and loved ones is essential in creating a tailored plan that addresses individual needs and preferences.

Use of Assistive Devices (Magnifiers, Large Print)

Assistive devices can significantly enhance the quality of life for individuals with vision loss. Magnifiers, for instance, come in various types, including handheld and electronic versions, which can help with reading small print or viewing details in images. When selecting a magnifier, consider factors such as the level of magnification needed and ease of use. Many devices are portable, making them convenient for use at home or on the go.

Large print materials are another valuable resource. This includes books, newspapers, and labels that feature bigger fonts, allowing for easier reading and comprehension. Many public libraries offer large print collections, and numerous online retailers provide options for purchasing large print books. Utilizing these devices and materials can empower individuals to maintain independence in daily activities, such as reading and crafting.

Importance of Support Groups and Community Resources

Support groups play a crucial role in helping individuals cope with vision loss by providing a platform for sharing experiences and strategies. Participating in these groups can foster a sense of community, reducing feelings of isolation and loneliness. Many groups offer meetings both in-person and online, making it easier to connect with others facing similar challenges. These connections can lead to valuable friendships and emotional support, enhancing overall well-being.

Community resources, such as local organizations dedicated to vision loss, can also provide essential services. These may include workshops on adaptive techniques, access to assistive technologies, and information about financial assistance. Researching available resources in your area can create a strong support network, enabling individuals to navigate their vision loss journey more effectively.

Counseling Services for Emotional Support

Counseling services offer valuable emotional support for individuals experiencing vision loss. These services can help address feelings of grief, anxiety, or depression that may arise from the changes in vision. A qualified counselor can provide coping strategies tailored to the individual's specific experiences and emotional needs, facilitating a healthier mental outlook.

Additionally, group therapy can be beneficial, as it allows individuals to share their stories in a supportive environment. Hearing others' experiences can validate feelings and inspire new coping techniques. When seeking counseling services, look for professionals who specialize in vision loss or chronic illness to ensure the most relevant support.

The Role of Family and Caregivers in Adaptation

Family members and caregivers are vital in helping individuals adapt to vision loss. Their support can include assisting with daily tasks, providing encouragement, and participating in educational programs about vision loss. Open communication between the individual and their support network is crucial, as it fosters understanding and ensures that needs are met effectively.

Encouraging independence is also essential; caregivers can help by offering assistance while allowing individuals to complete tasks on their own. This balance promotes confidence and self-esteem, which are vital for emotional well-being. Training family members in the use of assistive devices can further enhance their ability to support the individual's needs effectively.

Tips for Maintaining Independence at Home

Maintaining independence at home is achievable with thoughtful adjustments. One effective tip is to declutter living spaces, ensuring that pathways are clear and familiar objects are easy to locate. Organizing items consistently can reduce confusion and enhance navigation. Additionally, labeling important items with large print or Braille can help individuals find what they need without assistance.

Utilizing adaptive equipment, such as talking appliances or smart home technology, can further support independence. For instance, smart speakers can help with reminders and information without needing visual interaction. Regularly assessing the home environment for potential hazards and making necessary adjustments can also enhance safety and confidence in navigating the space independently.

Engaging in Hobbies and Activities with Vision Loss

Engaging in hobbies can bring joy and fulfillment despite vision loss. Finding activities that can be adapted, such as audio books, music, or tactile crafts, allows individuals to continue enjoying their passions. Many hobbies also provide opportunities for social interaction, which can enhance emotional well-being. Exploring local classes or community centers offering adaptive programs can open doors to new interests.

Adapting existing hobbies is another option. For example, cooking can involve using larger utensils or labeled containers, while gardening can include raised beds for easier access. Encouraging creativity and exploration in hobbies fosters a sense of accomplishment and provides a positive distraction from the challenges of vision loss.

Planning for Daily Activities and Tasks

Effective planning is essential for managing daily activities with vision loss. Creating a structured schedule can help prioritize tasks and ensure that important activities are not overlooked. Using planners with larger print or digital reminders can aid in organization and time management. Breaking tasks into smaller, manageable steps can also reduce overwhelm and increase productivity.

Involving family members in planning can provide additional support and help coordinate tasks. For example, delegating certain responsibilities or scheduling regular check-ins can foster collaboration and maintain a sense of community. Being flexible and willing to adapt plans as needed can enhance resilience and improve overall efficiency.

The Significance of Good Lighting in Living Spaces

Good lighting is crucial for individuals with vision loss. Proper illumination can enhance visibility and reduce strain on the eyes, making it easier to navigate spaces. Using adjustable lamps and strategically placing light sources can create a more comfortable environment. It is essential to consider the type of lighting as well; bright, direct light is often more effective than softer ambient lighting.

Eliminating glare is another important aspect of effective lighting. Using matte surfaces and positioning lights to avoid reflections can improve visibility. Regularly evaluating the lighting in different areas of the home and making adjustments can significantly impact comfort and independence in daily activities.

Accessibility Considerations in Home and Public Spaces

Accessibility is vital for individuals with vision loss to navigate their environments safely and independently. At home, implementing features such as handrails, non-slip mats, and clear pathways can enhance safety. It's beneficial to evaluate furniture placement to ensure that items are easily accessible and do not obstruct movement.

In public spaces, advocating for accessibility measures is crucial. This includes requesting features like tactile paths, Braille signage, and audio announcements in transportation systems. Engaging with local organizations that focus on disability rights can help promote awareness and push for necessary changes in community infrastructure.

Staying Socially Connected Despite Vision Challenges

Maintaining social connections is essential for emotional well-being, even with vision challenges. Scheduling regular phone calls or video chats with friends and family can help nurture these relationships. Additionally, exploring community events or clubs focused on shared interests can foster new friendships and support networks.

Engaging in online communities dedicated to vision loss can also provide a sense of belonging. Many platforms offer discussion forums, social media groups, and virtual events, allowing individuals to connect with others who share similar experiences. By leveraging technology and fostering in-person relationships, individuals can stay socially connected and supported.

Utilizing Technology for Assistance

Technology offers numerous solutions for managing vision loss. Screen readers and magnification software can enhance access to digital content, making it easier to read emails, browse the web, or use apps. Learning to utilize these tools can open up a world of information and opportunities for engagement.

Smartphone applications designed for the visually impaired can provide valuable assistance in daily life. For instance, apps that identify objects, read text aloud, or provide navigation support can enhance independence. Exploring various technologies and finding the right tools for individual needs can empower users to adapt to their circumstances effectively.

Personal Anecdotes and Success Stories

Personal anecdotes and success stories can serve as powerful sources of inspiration and motivation for individuals facing vision loss. Hearing how others have navigated their challenges and adapted their lives can provide practical insights and instill hope. Many organizations dedicated to vision loss share these stories through newsletters, websites, or community events.

Connecting with individuals who have experienced similar challenges can foster a sense of community and shared understanding. Engaging in discussions about overcoming obstacles and celebrating achievements can encourage resilience and reinforce the idea that a fulfilling life is possible despite vision loss.

CHAPTER 6:

Vision Preservation Strategies

Nutritional Tips for Eye Health

To maintain optimal eye health, focus on a balanced diet that includes plenty of fruits and vegetables. Foods rich in vitamins A, C, and E, along with zinc, can significantly contribute to good vision. Incorporating colorful fruits and vegetables, such as carrots, spinach, and bell peppers, ensures a robust intake of antioxidants, which protect the eyes from oxidative stress.

In addition to fruits and vegetables, consider adding whole grains and lean proteins to your meals. Whole grains contain essential nutrients that help maintain healthy blood sugar levels, which is particularly important for diabetic individuals. Regularly consuming a variety of food sources will provide your body with the nutrients it needs to support eye health.

Foods Rich in Lutein and Zeaxanthin

Lutein and zeaxanthin are powerful antioxidants found in high concentrations in dark leafy greens like kale, spinach, and collard greens. To maximize your intake, try to include at least one serving of these greens in your daily meals, whether through salads, smoothies, or cooked dishes. These nutrients help filter harmful blue light and reduce the risk of macular degeneration.

In addition to greens, other sources of lutein and zeaxanthin include broccoli, corn, and eggs. Incorporating these foods into your diet can be as simple as adding them to your omelets, stir-fries, or even snacks. Aim for a colorful plate to ensure you're getting a variety of these beneficial compounds.

The Importance of Omega-3 Fatty Acids

Omega-3 fatty acids are essential for maintaining retinal health and preventing dry eye syndrome. Rich sources of omega-3s include fatty fish such as salmon, mackerel, and sardines. Aim to eat fatty fish at least twice a week, or consider incorporating omega-3 supplements if you're vegetarian or allergic to fish.

Plant-based sources of omega-3s, such as flaxseeds, chia seeds, and walnuts, are also beneficial. You can sprinkle these seeds on yogurt, oatmeal, or salads to boost your intake easily. Including omega-3 fatty acids in your diet will help support overall eye health and reduce inflammation.

Regular Exercise and Its Benefits for Eye Health

Engaging in regular physical activity has numerous benefits, including improving blood circulation, which is crucial for eye health. Aim for at least 150 minutes of moderate exercise each week, such as brisk walking, cycling, or swimming. This not only benefits your cardiovascular health but also reduces the risk of diseases that can negatively impact vision.

In addition to cardiovascular exercise, incorporating strength training and flexibility exercises can enhance overall wellness. Activities like yoga and tai chi promote relaxation and may help alleviate symptoms of eye strain. Establish a routine that fits your lifestyle, making it easier to maintain consistency and improve your eye health.

Managing Other Health Conditions (e.g., Diabetes)

Managing health conditions like diabetes is vital for preserving eye health, as uncontrolled blood sugar levels can lead to diabetic retinopathy. Monitor your blood glucose levels regularly and work with your healthcare provider to create a management plan that includes medication, diet, and exercise. This proactive approach will help minimize the risk of complications related to vision.

Incorporate regular check-ups with your eye care professional to monitor any changes in your vision. Discuss any concerns with your doctor and ensure that they are aware of your medical history. By staying vigilant and managing your overall health, you can protect your vision and address any potential issues early.

Smoking Cessation Resources

Quitting smoking significantly reduces the risk of developing age-related eye diseases, including cataracts and macular degeneration. If you smoke, explore resources like counseling, support groups, or nicotine replacement therapies to assist with cessation. Many health organizations offer free resources that can guide you through the quitting process.

Set achievable goals and track your progress to stay motivated. Consider using apps or journaling to document your journey. Support from friends and family can also play a critical role, so share your goals with them and seek encouragement when needed.

Tips for Protecting Eyes from UV Rays

To protect your eyes from harmful UV rays, invest in sunglasses that block 100% of UVA and UVB rays. Look for sunglasses labeled with a UV protection rating, and make sure they fit well to provide full coverage. Wearing a wide-brimmed hat can further shield your eyes when outdoors.

Limit sun exposure during peak hours (10 a.m. to 4 p.m.) and seek shade whenever possible. Educate yourself on the importance of eye protection in different environments, such as at the beach or during winter sports, to ensure you're consistently safeguarding your vision from UV damage.

Strategies for Reducing Digital Eye Strain

To minimize digital eye strain, practice the 20-20-20 rule: every 20 minutes, take a 20-second break to look at something 20 feet away. This simple technique helps relax your eye muscles and reduces fatigue. Additionally, adjust your screen brightness and contrast to ensure comfort while using digital devices.

Creating a comfortable workspace can also help alleviate eye strain. Position your screen at eye level and about an arm's length away. Using blue light filters or glasses can further reduce glare from screens, enhancing your visual comfort during prolonged use.

Importance of Hydration for Overall Health

Staying hydrated is essential for maintaining overall health, including eye health. Dehydration can lead to dry eyes, which can cause discomfort and vision issues. Aim to drink at least eight 8-ounce glasses of water daily, adjusting your intake based on activity levels and climate.

Incorporating water-rich foods, such as cucumbers, oranges, and watermelon, can also contribute to your hydration goals. Monitor your body's signals for thirst and aim to keep a water bottle handy throughout the day, making it easier to maintain adequate hydration.

Mindfulness and Stress-Reduction Techniques

Practicing mindfulness and stress-reduction techniques can improve overall well-being, including eye health. Activities such as meditation, deep breathing exercises, and gentle yoga can help reduce stress levels. Dedicate a few minutes each day to engage in these practices, focusing on your breathing and clearing your mind.

Creating a calming environment can enhance your mindfulness practice. Designate a quiet space in your home where you can relax without distractions. Incorporate soothing elements, such as soft lighting and calming scents, to promote a peaceful atmosphere for relaxation.

The Role of Routine Eye Care

Regular eye examinations are crucial for maintaining eye health and detecting issues early. Schedule comprehensive eye exams at least once a year, even if you have no vision problems. An eye care professional can identify potential concerns and recommend appropriate treatments or lifestyle changes.

During your visit, discuss any changes in your vision and any concerns you may have. Adhering to your eye care provider's recommendations ensures that you're taking proactive steps to protect your vision and maintain your overall eye health.

Creating an Eye-Friendly Environment

Designing an eye-friendly environment involves optimizing lighting and reducing glare. Use soft, diffused lighting to minimize harsh reflections and eye strain. Consider installing adjustable blinds or curtains to control natural light, ensuring comfort during various times of the day.

Organize your living space to reduce clutter and improve organization, allowing you to navigate your environment safely. Incorporate plants or decorative items that can enhance your mood while promoting a calming atmosphere, contributing positively to your eye health.

Regular Monitoring and Adjustments in Lifestyle

Consistently monitor your vision and make adjustments to your lifestyle as needed. Keep a log of any changes in your eyesight or discomfort you may experience. This information can be valuable during your eye exams, helping your eye care provider to make informed recommendations.

Incorporate regular evaluations of your diet, exercise routines, and overall health practices. Stay informed about new findings in eye health and adapt your habits to align with the best recommendations. By being proactive, you can ensure that your lifestyle choices are supporting your vision health over time.

CHAPTER 7:

Lifestyle Adjustments for Better Vision

Adapting Living Spaces for Visual Comfort

Creating a visually comfortable living environment is essential for individuals experiencing vision loss. Start by maximizing natural light in your home; use sheer curtains or blinds that can be adjusted to let in more sunlight. Arrange furniture to provide clear pathways and minimize obstacles, ensuring adequate space for movement. Utilize contrasting colors for walls, furniture, and decor to help differentiate objects and reduce visual confusion.

Additionally, incorporate adjustable lighting options, such as dimmers and task lighting, to enhance visibility in different areas of your home. Consider using large-print labels or tactile markers on frequently used items and appliances to make them easier to identify.

Regularly reassess your living space to ensure it continues to meet your visual comfort needs.

Importance of Routine Eye Examinations

Routine eye examinations are crucial for early detection of macular degeneration and other eye conditions. Schedule comprehensive eye exams with an eye care professional at least once a year, or more frequently if recommended based on your individual risk factors. During these exams, your eye doctor will assess your vision, check for any changes in your eyes, and discuss potential treatment options if needed.

Understanding the importance of these check-ups can empower you to take charge of your eye health. Make it a habit to keep a calendar or reminder system for your appointments, and consider bringing a family member or friend for support, especially if you have concerns about traveling to and from the appointment.

Setting Up a Vision-Friendly Workspace

To create a vision-friendly workspace, start by optimizing lighting. Use natural light where possible and consider adjustable lamps with bright, white light to illuminate your work area without causing glare. Position your computer screen at eye level and about an arm's length away to reduce strain on your eyes. Additionally, use large fonts and high-contrast colors for text on your screen to improve readability.

Organize your workspace to reduce clutter, making it easier to find necessary items. Consider using tools such as magnifiers or text-to-speech software to assist with reading documents. Regularly take breaks to rest your eyes, and practice the 20-20-20 rule: every 20 minutes, look at something 20 feet away for at least 20 seconds to help alleviate eye strain.

Engaging in Community Resources and Activities

Getting involved in community resources can provide valuable support and social interaction for those with vision loss. Research local organizations or support groups that focus on vision health, as they often offer programs, workshops, and events tailored to individuals with macular degeneration. Attending these activities can help you meet others with similar experiences and share coping strategies.

Many communities also provide services like transportation assistance and vision rehabilitation programs. Reach out to local health departments or vision centers to find out what resources are available. Taking advantage of these services not only enhances your quality of life but also encourages active participation in your community.

How to Effectively Communicate Vision Needs

Effectively communicating your vision needs is crucial for receiving the support you require. Start by being open about your vision challenges with family, friends, and coworkers. Use clear language to describe how your vision impairment affects daily tasks, and don't hesitate to ask for specific accommodations, such as better lighting or assistance with navigation in unfamiliar environments.

In professional settings, consider providing information about your visual needs to your employer or HR department. Many workplaces have policies in place to support employees with disabilities, including vision loss. By advocating for yourself, you empower others to understand your situation and assist you more effectively.

Planning Travel and Outdoor Activities with Vision Loss

Planning travel and outdoor activities with vision loss requires careful consideration and preparation. Before heading out, familiarize yourself with the environment using tools such as maps, GPS applications, or even descriptions from friends. Consider bringing along a sighted companion who can help navigate and provide assistance as needed, ensuring a smoother experience.

Also, explore accessible transportation options in your area, like public transit services that accommodate individuals with disabilities. When participating in outdoor activities, choose well-lit and familiar locations, and be mindful of your surroundings. Inform your travel companions of your vision needs to ensure everyone is on the same page and prepared for any potential challenges.

Strategies for Cooking and Food Preparation

Cooking with vision loss can be safely managed by implementing a few practical strategies. Start by organizing your kitchen to ensure that frequently used items are within easy reach and labeled clearly. Use contrasting colors for kitchen tools, like cutting boards and utensils, to help distinguish between them. Invest in adaptive tools such as measuring cups with large markings or talking kitchen scales.

While cooking, focus on sensory cues, such as smells and sounds, to gauge the readiness of food. You can also use tactile markers on stove dials and oven knobs to differentiate between settings. Practicing these techniques will build your confidence in the kitchen, allowing you to prepare meals independently and safely.

Importance of Maintaining a Healthy Weight

Maintaining a healthy weight is crucial for overall health and can significantly impact vision health. Start by focusing on a balanced diet rich in fruits, vegetables, whole grains, and lean proteins. Limit your intake of saturated fats, sugars, and processed foods. Keeping a food diary can help track your daily intake and promote healthier choices.

Incorporating regular physical activity into your routine is equally important. Aim for at least 150 minutes of moderate aerobic activity each week, such as walking or swimming. Engaging in physical activities not only helps manage weight but also improves overall well-being, making it easier to cope with vision-related challenges.

Coping with Vision-Related Stressors

Coping with vision-related stressors involves developing effective strategies to manage anxiety and frustration associated with vision loss. Start by acknowledging your feelings and giving yourself permission to grieve the changes in your vision. Consider engaging in mindfulness practices, such as meditation or deep-breathing exercises, to promote relaxation and reduce stress.

Additionally, seek support from friends, family, or support groups who understand your experience. Sharing your feelings and challenges with others can provide emotional relief and practical advice. Don't hesitate to explore professional counseling if you find it difficult to manage stress on your own, as mental health is just as vital as physical health.

Staying Informed About Community Programs

Staying informed about community programs can greatly benefit individuals dealing with vision loss. Subscribe to newsletters or follow local organizations on social media to receive updates about workshops, health fairs, and support groups in your area. Many organizations offer resources for navigating vision challenges and enhancing quality of life.

Attend community meetings or events to network with other individuals facing similar challenges. This engagement can help you stay updated on available services and programs, such as transportation assistance or vision rehabilitation workshops. Being proactive about seeking information allows you to make informed decisions about your care and support options.

Building a Supportive Network of Friends and Family

Building a supportive network is essential for coping with vision loss. Start by openly communicating your needs and challenges to friends and family members. Encourage them to participate in activities that can accommodate your vision impairment, such as hosting gatherings in well-lit environments or discussing any necessary adjustments for outings.

Additionally, consider joining support groups or community organizations where you can connect with others who understand your experiences. Engaging with like-minded individuals can provide a sense of camaraderie and shared understanding, fostering a stronger support system that encourages emotional well-being.

Participating in Vision Health Advocacy

Participating in vision health advocacy allows you to raise awareness about the challenges faced by individuals with vision loss. Start by educating yourself on issues affecting the visually impaired community and engaging in local advocacy efforts, such as attending town hall meetings or joining advocacy groups focused on eye health.

You can also share your story through social media or local events to highlight the importance of eye health and early detection. Your voice can inspire others to take action and seek necessary resources, creating a more supportive environment for individuals experiencing vision loss.

Monitoring Personal Vision Changes Over Time

Monitoring your personal vision changes over time is crucial for managing macular degeneration. Keep a log of any noticeable changes in your vision, such as blurriness or difficulty seeing at certain distances. Regularly assess your vision using an Amsler grid, which can help detect any new distortions or changes in your central vision.

Communicate any significant changes to your eye care professional during routine examinations. Being proactive about monitoring your vision enables early detection of potential complications, allowing for timely interventions and adjustments to your treatment plan.

CHAPTER 8:

Common Concerns about Macular Degeneration

Addressing Fears of Vision Loss

Fears surrounding vision loss can be overwhelming, but acknowledging these fears is the first step toward managing them. Individuals can benefit from seeking support through counseling or support groups, where they can express their concerns and hear from others who are facing similar challenges. Engaging in discussions with healthcare professionals can also provide clarity about the condition and reassure individuals about the measures available for vision preservation.

Practical steps include educating oneself about macular degeneration and its potential outcomes, which can help demystify the condition. Understanding that while some vision loss may occur, many people can maintain significant levels of sight and quality of life with appropriate strategies and treatments. This knowledge can empower individuals to take proactive steps toward managing their eye health.

Myths vs. Reality about Treatments

There are many myths about treatments for macular degeneration that can lead to confusion and unnecessary anxiety. One common myth is that there is a single "cure" for the condition, when in reality, treatment often involves a combination of lifestyle changes, medications, and therapies tailored to the individual's specific needs. Understanding the actual options available—such as injections, laser treatments, and nutritional supplements—can help set realistic expectations.

To combat misinformation, individuals should consult reputable sources, such as eye care professionals or validated health organizations. Keeping up with the latest research and treatment developments can also provide hope and guidance. Engaging in discussions with healthcare providers can further clarify treatment plans and empower individuals to make informed decisions about their care.

Concerns Regarding Lifestyle Changes

Lifestyle changes can feel daunting for those diagnosed with macular degeneration, but they are essential for managing the condition. Simple modifications, such as incorporating more leafy greens and omega-3 fatty acids into the diet, can help support eye health. Regular exercise is also beneficial; activities like walking or swimming improve circulation and overall well-being, contributing to better vision outcomes.

It's helpful to approach these lifestyle changes gradually. Setting small, achievable goals, such as adding one serving of vegetables to meals each day or committing to short daily walks, can make the transition feel less overwhelming. Joining a cooking class focused on healthy meals or a local walking group can also provide motivation and support while making these changes more enjoyable.

The Impact of Macular Degeneration on Mental Health

Macular degeneration can significantly affect mental health, leading to feelings of anxiety and depression. The fear of losing independence and the ability to perform daily tasks can be particularly distressing. It's important for individuals to recognize these emotional responses and seek help through therapy or support groups, which can provide a safe space to share experiences and feelings.

Incorporating mindfulness practices, such as meditation or yoga, can also be beneficial in managing stress and anxiety related to vision loss. These practices encourage relaxation and help individuals maintain a positive outlook. Keeping a journal to express thoughts and emotions can serve as a therapeutic outlet, further supporting mental well-being during challenging times.

Managing Financial Concerns
Related to Treatment

Financial concerns related to treatment for macular degeneration can be significant and stressful. Individuals should begin by consulting with their healthcare providers to understand the costs associated with their specific treatment plans. Many facilities offer financial counseling or assistance programs that can help navigate insurance coverage and out-of-pocket expenses.

Additionally, exploring resources such as community health programs, non-profit organizations, and government assistance can provide further support. These resources may offer information about subsidies or grants for vision-related expenses. Creating a budget that includes potential treatment costs and discussing options with family members can also alleviate some financial pressure.

Questions About the Safety of Supplements

Many people consider dietary supplements to support their eye health but may have concerns about their safety and efficacy. It's important to consult with a healthcare professional before starting any supplement regimen, as they can provide guidance based on individual health needs and potential interactions with medications. Researching supplements with proven benefits for macular degeneration, such as lutein and zeaxanthin, can also be beneficial.

When choosing supplements, look for those that have been tested and approved by recognized organizations. Checking for third-party certifications can ensure quality and safety. Keeping a log of any changes experienced after starting a supplement can help in discussions with healthcare providers, ensuring that any necessary adjustments can be made.

Addressing Family Members' Fears and Concerns

Family members often experience their own fears and concerns regarding a loved one's vision loss. Open communication is vital; discussing feelings and anxieties about macular degeneration can help family members understand the condition better and feel more involved in the care process. Sharing educational materials about the disease can also provide clarity and dispel misconceptions.

Encouraging family members to participate in appointments with healthcare providers can further alleviate concerns. This involvement allows them to ask questions and gain firsthand knowledge about the condition and treatment options. Creating a supportive environment where everyone can express their feelings and share resources fosters a stronger family bond during challenging times.

Understanding the Progression of the Disease

Understanding the progression of macular degeneration can help individuals prepare for changes in vision. Typically, the disease may progress slowly, with early stages often showing few noticeable symptoms. Regular eye examinations are crucial, as they can help monitor changes and identify when treatment or interventions are necessary.

Educating oneself about the signs of progression, such as difficulty recognizing faces or reading, can facilitate timely intervention. Keeping a log of vision changes can also be beneficial during doctor visits. This proactive approach enables individuals to make informed decisions about their care and maintain a sense of control over their condition.

The Role of Healthcare Providers in Easing Concerns

Healthcare providers play a vital role in easing concerns related to macular degeneration. They are essential for providing accurate information about the condition and available treatments. Regular check-ups allow healthcare professionals to monitor the progression of the disease and adjust treatment plans as needed, helping patients feel more secure in their care.

Patients should feel empowered to ask questions and express their concerns during appointments. Building a rapport with healthcare providers can foster trust and improve communication, ensuring that individuals receive comprehensive support. Participating in educational workshops or seminars hosted by eye care professionals can also enhance understanding and ease concerns.

Importance of Education and Information

Education about macular degeneration is essential for effective management of the condition. Understanding the disease's nature, potential progression, and available treatments enables individuals to make informed decisions about their health. Seeking reliable information from trusted sources, such as medical professionals and reputable organizations, can enhance knowledge and preparedness.

Creating a personal information toolkit, including brochures, articles, and educational videos, can provide ongoing resources for reference. Attending support groups and community events focused on eye health can also facilitate learning and help individuals feel connected to others facing similar challenges.

Connecting with Others Facing Similar Challenges

Connecting with others who are experiencing similar challenges can provide invaluable emotional support. Participating in support groups, either in-person or online, allows individuals to share their experiences, exchange tips, and gain insights into managing macular degeneration. These connections can foster a sense of community and reduce feelings of isolation.

Social media platforms and dedicated forums are great places to find and join such groups. Sharing personal stories and listening to others can promote understanding and resilience, helping individuals navigate their journey with macular degeneration together.

Strategies for Open Communication with Loved Ones

Open communication with loved ones about macular degeneration is crucial for support and understanding.

Initiating conversations about feelings and concerns related to vision loss can help family and friends provide the necessary emotional and practical support. Setting aside time to discuss these topics can strengthen relationships and enhance mutual understanding.

Using clear language and being specific about needs can facilitate more productive conversations. Encourage loved ones to ask questions and express their concerns, creating a two-way dialogue. Regularly checking in with each other can help maintain open lines of communication as the situation evolves.

Importance of Celebrating Small Victories in Vision Care

Celebrating small victories in vision care can significantly boost morale and motivation. Whether it's successfully adapting to a new treatment or making healthier lifestyle choices, recognizing these achievements fosters a positive outlook. Keeping a journal of these milestones can serve as a reminder of progress made, even amidst challenges.

Involving family and friends in these celebrations can enhance the sense of accomplishment. Sharing successes with loved ones not only reinforces support networks but also encourages continued efforts in managing macular degeneration effectively. These small victories can make a big difference in maintaining hope and motivation.

CHAPTER 9:

FAQs about Macular Degeneration

What are the early signs of macular degeneration?

Early signs of macular degeneration may include blurred or distorted vision, especially when looking at straight lines, which can appear wavy or bent. You might also notice difficulty in recognizing faces or a gradual loss of color vision. Spotting these changes early is crucial as they can indicate the onset of age-related macular degeneration (AMD), allowing for timely intervention.

To monitor your vision, consider using an Amsler grid, a simple tool that helps detect vision changes. By looking at the grid and noting any distortions or missing areas, you can keep track of your visual health and share any concerns with your eye care professional promptly.

How is macular degeneration diagnosed?

Macular degeneration is diagnosed through a comprehensive eye examination that includes visual acuity tests, dilated eye exams, and imaging tests like optical coherence tomography (OCT). During the dilated exam, the doctor uses drops to widen your pupils and then examines the retina for any changes or damage to the macula.

If AMD is suspected, your eye doctor may also perform a fluoresce in angiography, which involves injecting a dye into your bloodstream and taking pictures of the blood vessels in your eye. This helps to assess the extent of the condition and determine the most appropriate treatment options.

What treatments are available for macular degeneration?

Treatment options for macular degeneration vary based on the type and severity of the condition. For wet AMD, which involves abnormal blood vessel growth, anti-VEGF injections are commonly used to inhibit further growth and leakage. These treatments can help maintain vision and, in some cases, improve it.

For dry AMD, there are currently no FDA-approved treatments, but certain dietary supplements may slow progression. Nutritional approaches, such as the AREDS2 formulation containing vitamins C and E, zinc, and lutein, can support eye health. Regular monitoring by your eye care professional is essential to track changes and manage any progression.

Is macular degeneration hereditary?

Yes, genetic factors play a significant role in macular degeneration. Research indicates that individuals with a family history of AMD are at a higher risk of developing the condition themselves. Specific genes have been identified that are linked to increased susceptibility to AMD, emphasizing the importance of family health history in understanding your risk.

To assess your risk, discuss your family history with your eye doctor, who may recommend earlier and more frequent screenings if you have close relatives with AMD. Genetic testing is also available for those interested in understanding their individual risk further.

Can diet really make a difference in eye health?

Absolutely! A diet rich in antioxidants, vitamins, and omega-3 fatty acids can significantly contribute to eye health and may reduce the risk of developing macular degeneration. Foods like leafy greens (spinach, kale), colorful fruits (berries, oranges), and fish (salmon, sardines) are particularly beneficial.

To incorporate these foods into your diet, aim for a colorful plate at every meal. Consider adding a salad with dark greens and orange peppers, or include fatty fish in your weekly menu to support your overall eye health and potentially slow the progression of AMD.

What lifestyle changes can help preserve vision?

Making certain lifestyle changes can play a vital role in preserving vision and managing macular degeneration. Quitting smoking, maintaining a healthy weight, and exercising regularly can reduce your risk of AMD progression. These changes not only benefit your eyes but also enhance your overall well-being.

Additionally, protecting your eyes from UV light is crucial. Wearing sunglasses with UV protection when outdoors can help safeguard your vision. Establishing a routine of regular eye exams can help detect any changes early, allowing for timely interventions.

How often should I have my eyes examined?

The frequency of eye examinations depends on your age, health status, and risk factors for macular degeneration. Generally, adults over 60 should have comprehensive eye exams at least once a year. If you have risk factors such as a family history of AMD or existing vision problems, more frequent visits may be necessary.

To ensure you stay on track, schedule your appointments ahead of time and keep a calendar of your eye exams. This proactive approach helps maintain your eye health and allows for early detection of any changes in your vision.

Are there support groups for people with macular degeneration?

Yes, numerous support groups and organizations exist to assist individuals with macular degeneration. These groups offer a platform for sharing experiences, gaining emotional support, and learning practical strategies to cope with vision loss. Organizations like the American Macular Degeneration Foundation provide valuable resources and community connections.

To find a support group, start by checking local community centers or hospitals for resources. Online platforms and social media can also connect you with virtual support networks, allowing you to engage with others facing similar challenges.

What assistive devices are available for those with vision loss?

Several assistive devices can help individuals with vision loss maintain independence and improve their quality of life. Common options include magnifying glasses, handheld magnifiers, and digital magnifying devices, which can enhance reading and everyday tasks. Additionally, screen readers and text-to-speech software can assist in accessing digital content.

To explore these options, visit your local optometrist or an organization specializing in vision loss rehabilitation. They can recommend specific devices tailored to your needs and offer training on how to use them effectively in daily life.

How can I cope with emotional challenges related to vision loss?

Coping with emotional challenges due to vision loss involves acknowledging your feelings and seeking support. It's essential to talk about your emotions with friends, family, or a counselor, as expressing your thoughts can alleviate stress and anxiety. Finding a support group, as mentioned earlier, can also provide an outlet for sharing experiences and receiving encouragement from others.

Additionally, engaging in activities you enjoy can help improve your mood and provide a sense of normalcy. Whether it's pursuing hobbies, volunteering, or connecting with friends, staying active and involved can enhance your emotional well-being during this challenging time.

What are the latest advancements in macular degeneration research?

Recent advancements in macular degeneration research focus on new treatments and preventive measures. Ongoing clinical trials are exploring novel therapies, including gene therapy and new anti-VEGF agents that could improve outcomes for patients with wet AMD. These developments aim to enhance vision preservation and potentially restore sight in those affected by the disease.

To stay updated on the latest research findings, consider subscribing to newsletters from reputable eye health organizations or following academic journals specializing in ophthalmology. Engaging with research news can help you remain informed about potential treatment options and advancements in care.

How can family and friends help someone with macular degeneration?

Family and friends play a crucial role in supporting individuals with macular degeneration. They can assist by offering emotional support, helping with daily tasks, and encouraging the use of assistive devices. Providing a listening ear and understanding the challenges faced can significantly improve the individual's quality of life.

Additionally, family members can help by accompanying their loved ones to eye appointments, assisting in organizing medications, and advocating for them in healthcare settings. This support can alleviate stress and foster a collaborative environment focused on managing the condition together.

Where can I find more information and resources on macular degeneration?

Finding reliable information and resources on macular degeneration is essential for effective management. Start by visiting reputable organizations such as the American Academy of Ophthalmology or the National Eye Institute, which offer comprehensive guides on the condition, treatment options, and support networks.

Local libraries, hospitals, and community health centers can also provide literature and referrals to educational programs or support groups. Utilizing these resources can empower you with knowledge and a sense of community as you navigate the challenges of macular degeneration.

Conclusion

Maintaining eye health begins with regular eye examinations. These exams can help detect early signs of macular degeneration and other eye conditions. It's advisable to have comprehensive eye exams every one to two years, especially if you're over 50 or have risk factors such as a family history of eye diseases. During these exams, your eye care professional will check for changes in your vision and the health of your retina.

In addition to regular check-ups, adopting a healthy lifestyle can contribute significantly to eye health. This includes eating a balanced diet rich in fruits, vegetables, and omega-3 fatty acids, as well as maintaining a healthy weight. Protecting your eyes from harmful UV rays by wearing sunglasses and avoiding smoking are also crucial steps in preserving eye health.

Early Detection

Early detection of macular degeneration is vital for managing the condition effectively. Regular screenings using tests such as the Amsler grid can help you notice any changes in your central vision early on. If you notice blurred or distorted vision, it's essential to consult an eye care professional immediately.

Advanced imaging techniques, like optical coherence tomography (OCT), can provide detailed images of the retina, allowing for precise diagnosis. The earlier the condition is detected, the more options there are for management and treatment, potentially slowing the progression of the disease.

Treatment Options

There are several treatment options for managing macular degeneration. For dry macular degeneration, no specific treatment exists, but nutritional supplements containing vitamins C and E, zinc, and lutein may slow its progression. For wet macular degeneration, treatments like anti-VEGF injections can reduce the growth of abnormal blood vessels and preserve vision.

Laser therapy is another option, which can help seal leaking blood vessels in the eye. It's essential to discuss these treatment options with your eye care provider to determine the most suitable plan based on your specific condition and lifestyle.

Risk Factors

Understanding the risk factors associated with macular degeneration can help you take preventative measures. Major risk factors include age, family history, smoking, obesity, and prolonged exposure to sunlight. Identifying these factors allows you to make informed decisions about your eye health.

To mitigate these risks, consider lifestyle changes like quitting smoking, managing weight, and practicing sun safety. Regular physical activity and a diet high in leafy greens and fish can also lower your risk of developing macular degeneration.

Improving Quality of Life

Improving the quality of life for those with macular degeneration involves utilizing tools and resources designed for low vision. Magnifying glasses, text-to-speech software, and specialized lighting can enhance reading and everyday activities. Learning to use these aids can significantly boost independence and confidence.

Support groups and counseling can also play a vital role in coping with the emotional impact of vision loss. Connecting with others who understand your challenges can provide comfort, practical advice, and encouragement to adapt to changing vision.

Vision Preservation Strategies

To preserve vision and slow the progression of macular degeneration, consider incorporating specific strategies into your daily routine. Regular exercise, such as walking or swimming, can improve overall health and circulation, benefiting eye health. Additionally, ensuring that your home is well-lit and reducing glare can help manage symptoms.

Implementing visual rehabilitation techniques, such as contrast sensitivity training, can also enhance your ability to see in different lighting conditions.

Collaborating with vision specialists can provide personalized strategies tailored to your specific needs.

Lifestyle Adjustments

Making lifestyle adjustments is crucial for managing macular degeneration effectively. Focus on maintaining a balanced diet, emphasizing fruits, vegetables, and whole grains while reducing processed foods and sugars. Staying hydrated and limiting alcohol consumption can further promote eye health.

Incorporating daily routines such as stretching and exercises tailored to improve eye strength can also be beneficial. Additionally, scheduling regular breaks from screens can reduce eye strain, helping to maintain visual comfort and health over time.

Nutritional Supplements

Nutritional supplements can play a significant role in managing macular degeneration. Research suggests that certain vitamins, such as A, C, E, and minerals like zinc and copper, may help slow the progression of the disease. Discussing with your healthcare provider about incorporating these supplements into your routine is advisable.

In addition to supplements, including foods rich in antioxidants, like leafy greens and colorful fruits, can enhance your diet. Omega-3 fatty acids found in fish like salmon and walnuts can also be beneficial for eye health, providing an additional layer of protection against degeneration.

Low Vision Rehabilitation

Low vision rehabilitation programs are designed to help individuals adapt to vision loss. These programs often include personalized training in the use of assistive devices and techniques to maximize remaining vision. Working with an occupational therapist can help you develop strategies for daily living activities.

Techniques such as using high-contrast colors, organizing spaces for easier navigation, and practicing visual skills can improve functionality and independence. Engaging in low vision support groups can also offer encouragement and practical tips from others facing similar challenges.

Vision-Friendly Environment

Creating a vision-friendly environment is essential for those with macular degeneration. This involves optimizing lighting conditions in your home, using soft, glare-free light sources, and ensuring adequate illumination in workspaces. Arranging furniture to minimize obstacles can help enhance mobility and safety.

Additionally, consider using visual cues, such as brightly colored tape on stairs or doorways, to improve spatial awareness. Implementing these changes can significantly enhance comfort and confidence in your daily activities, making life easier for those with vision impairment.

Support and Resources

Accessing support and resources is crucial for those affected by macular degeneration. Numerous organizations and online communities offer information, emotional support, and resources for coping with vision loss. Connecting with local or national groups can provide valuable insights and encouragement.

Many eye care professionals also offer resources, including brochures, workshops, and referral services, to help navigate available options. Utilizing these support systems can empower individuals and families to manage the impact of macular degeneration effectively.

Ongoing Research

Ongoing research into macular degeneration is crucial for discovering new treatment options and management strategies. Clinical trials are continuously being conducted to evaluate potential therapies, including gene therapy and stem cell treatments. Staying informed about these advancements can provide hope for better outcomes in the future.

Participating in research studies or trials may also be an option for individuals looking to contribute to the scientific understanding of macular degeneration. Engaging with the latest findings can inspire proactive approaches to managing vision loss and enhance the overall understanding of the condition.

Future Advancements

The future of macular degeneration treatment holds promise with advancements in technology and research. Innovations in imaging techniques and targeted therapies are paving the way for earlier detection and more effective management of the disease. Keeping up with the latest advancements can empower individuals to advocate for their eye health.

Furthermore, the development of wearable technology designed to assist with low vision is on the rise. These advancements can provide valuable tools for enhancing daily living, ultimately improving the quality of life for those affected by macular degeneration.